Cancer Control
Knowledge into Action
WHO Guide for Effective Programmes

Prevention

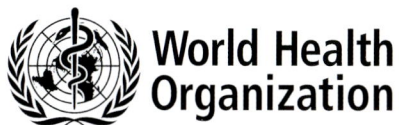

WHO Library Cataloguing-in-Publication Data

Prevention.
(Cancer control : knowledge into action : WHO guide for effective programmes ; module 2.)
1.Neoplasms – prevention and control. 2.Health planning. 3.National health programs – organization and administration. 4.Health policy. 5.Guidelines. I.World Health Organization. II.Series.
ISBN 92 4 154711 1   (NLM classification: QZ 200)

© World Health Organization 2007

All rights reserved. Publications of the World Health Organization can be obtained from WHO Press, World Health Organization, 20 Avenue Appia, 1211 Geneva 27, Switzerland (tel.: +41 22 791 3264; fax: +41 22 791 4857; e-mail: bookorders@who.int). Requests for permission to reproduce or translate WHO publications – whether for sale or for noncommercial distribution – should be addressed to WHO Press, at the above address (fax: +41 22 791 4806; e-mail: permissions@who.int).
The designations employed and the presentation of the material in this publication do not imply the expression of any opinion whatsoever on the part of the World Health Organization concerning the legal status of any country, territory, city or area or of its authorities, or concerning the delimitation of its frontiers or boundaries. Dotted lines on maps represent approximate border lines for which there may not yet be full agreement.
The mention of specific companies or of certain manufacturers' products does not imply that they are endorsed or recommended by the World Health Organization in preference to others of a similar nature that are not mentioned. Errors and omissions excepted, the names of proprietary products are distinguished by initial capital letters.
All reasonable precautions have been taken by the World Health Organization to verify the information contained in this publication. However, the published material is being distributed without warranty of any kind, either expressed or implied. The responsibility for the interpretation and use of the material lies with the reader. In no event shall the World Health Organization be liable for damages arising from its use.

The Prevention module of the Cancer Control Series is a joint effort of the following departments at WHO headquarters:

Chronic Diseases and Health Promotion; Ethics, Trade, Human Rights and Law; Immunization, Vaccines and Biologicals; Immunization, Vaccines and Research; Measurement and Health Information Systems; Mental Health and Substance Dependence; Public Health and Environment and the Tobacco Free Initiative; and also the WHO International Agency for Research on Cancer, Lyon, France.

The Prevention module was produced under the direction of Catherine Le Galès-Camus (Assistant Director-General, Noncommunicable Diseases and Mental Health), Robert Beaglehole (Director, Chronic Diseases and Health Promotion), Serge Resnikoff (Coordinator, Chronic Diseases Prevention and Management) and Cecilia Sepúlveda (Chronic Diseases Prevention and Management, coordinator of the overall series of modules).

Andreas Ullrich (Chronic Diseases Prevention and Management) was the coordinator for this module and provided extensive editorial input.

Editorial support was provided by Anthony Miller (scientific editor), Inés Salas (technical adviser), Angela Haden (technical writer and editor) and Paul Garwood (copy editor). Proofreading was done by Ann Morgan.

The production of the module was coordinated by Maria Villanueva.

Core contributions for the module were received from the following WHO staff:

Teresa Aguado, Antero Aitio, Timothy Armstrong, Annemieke Brands, Alexander Capron, Zhanat Carr, Felicity Cutts, Poonam Dhavan, JoAnne Epping-Jordan, Kathleen Irwin, Ivan Dimov Ivanov, Ingrid Keller, Colin Mathers, Yumiko Mochizuki, Isidore Obot, Armando Peruga, Vladimir Poznyak, Eva Rehfuss, Dag Rekve, Heide Richter-Airijoki, Craig Shapiro, Kurt Straif (IARC), Kate Strong, Angelika Tritscher, Colin Tukuitonga, Andreas Ullrich, Emilie van Deventer, Steven Wiersma and Hajo Zeeb.

Valuable input, help and advice were received from a number of people in WHO headquarters throughout the production of the module: Caroline Allsopp, David Bramley, Raphaël Crettaz, Maryvonne Grisetti and Rebecca Harding.

Cancer experts worldwide, as well as technical staff in WHO headquarters and in WHO regional and country offices, also provided valuable input by making contributions and reviewing the module, and are listed in the Acknowledgements.

Design and layout: This document's design is based on the Chronic Diseases and Health Promotion Department Style Guide developed by Reda Sadki, Paris, France. Further design and layout by L'IV Com Sàrl, Morges, Switzerland.

Printed in Switzerland

More information about this publication can be obtained from:
Department of Chronic Diseases and Health Promotion
World Health Organization
CH-1211 Geneva 27, Switzerland

The production of this publication was made possible through the generous financial support of the National Cancer Institute (NCI), USA, and the National Cancer Institute (Institut national du cancer, INCa), France. We would also like to thank the Public Health Agency of Canada (PHAC), the National Cancer Center of Korea (NCC), the International Atomic Energy Agency (IAEA) and the International Union Against Cancer (UICC) for their financial support.

Series overview

Introduction to the
Cancer Control Series

Cancer is to a large extent avoidable. Many cancers can be prevented. Others can be detected early in their development, treated and cured. Even with late stage cancer, the pain can be reduced, the progression of the cancer slowed, and patients and their families helped to cope.

Cancer is a leading cause of death globally. The World Health Organization estimates that 7.6 million people died of cancer in 2005 and 84 million people will die in the next 10 years if action is not taken. More than 70% of all cancer deaths occur in low- and middle-income countries, where resources available for prevention, diagnosis and treatment of cancer are limited or nonexistent.

But because of the wealth of available knowledge, all countries can, at some useful level, implement the four basic components of cancer control – *prevention, early detection, diagnosis and treatment, and palliative care* – and thus avoid and cure many cancers, as well as palliating the suffering.

Cancer control: knowledge into action, WHO guide for effective programmes is a series of six modules that provides practical advice for programme managers and policy-makers on how to advocate, plan and implement effective cancer control programmes, particularly in low- and middle-income countries.

A series of six modules

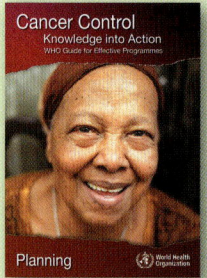

PLANNING
A practical guide for programme managers on how to plan overall cancer control effectively, according to available resources and integrating cancer control with programmes for other chronic diseases and related problems.

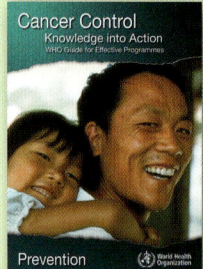

PREVENTION
a practical guide for programme managers on how to implement effective cancer prevention by controlling major avoidable cancer risk factors.

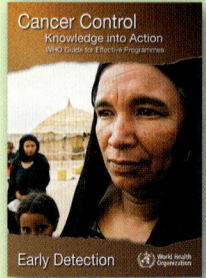

EARLY DETECTION
A practical guide for programme managers on how to implement effective early detection of major types of cancer that are amenable to early diagnosis and screening.

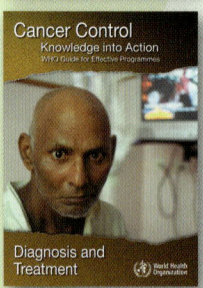

DIAGNOSIS AND TREATMENT
A practical guide for programme managers on how to implement effective cancer diagnosis and treatment, particularly linked to early detection programmes or curable cancers.

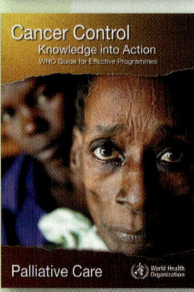

PALLIATIVE CARE
A practical guide for programme managers on how to implement effective palliative care for cancer, with a particular focus on community-based care.

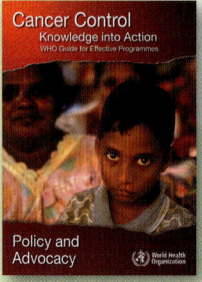

POLICY AND ADVOCACY
A practical guide for medium level decision-makers and programme managers on how to advocate for policy development and effective programme implementation for cancer control.

The WHO guide is a response to the World Health Assembly resolution on cancer prevention and control (WHA58.22), adopted in May 2005, which calls on Member States to intensify action against cancer by developing and reinforcing cancer control programmes. It builds on *National cancer control programmes: policies and managerial guidelines* and *Preventing chronic diseases: a vital investment*, as well as on the various WHO policies that have influenced efforts to control cancer.

Cancer control aims to reduce the incidence, morbidity and mortality of cancer and to improve the quality of life of cancer patients in a defined population, through the systematic implementation of evidence-based interventions for prevention, early detection, diagnosis, treatment, and palliative care. Comprehensive cancer control addresses the whole population, while seeking to respond to the needs of the different subgroups at risk.

COMPONENTS OF CANCER CONTROL

Prevention of cancer, especially when integrated with the prevention of chronic diseases and other related problems (such as reproductive health, hepatitis B immunization, HIV/AIDS, occupational and environmental health), offers the greatest public health potential and the most cost-effective long-term method of cancer control. We now have sufficient knowledge to prevent around 40% of all cancers. Most cancers are linked to tobacco use, unhealthy diet, or infectious agents (see Prevention module).

Early detection detects (or diagnoses) the disease at an early stage, when it has a high potential for cure (e.g. cervical or breast cancer). Interventions are available which permit the early detection and effective treatment of around one third of cases (see Early Detection module).

There are two strategies for early detection:
- *early diagnosis*, often involving the patient's awareness of early signs and symptoms, leading to a consultation with a health provider – who then promptly refers the patient for confirmation of diagnosis and treatment;
- *national or regional screening* of asymptomatic and apparently healthy individuals to detect pre-cancerous lesions or an early stage of cancer, and to arrange referral for diagnosis and treatment.

Series overview

Treatment aims to cure disease, prolong life, and improve the quality of remaining life after the diagnosis of cancer is confirmed by the appropriate available procedures. The most effective and efficient treatment is linked to early detection programmes and follows evidence-based standards of care. Patients can benefit either by cure or by prolonged life, in cases of cancers that although disseminated are highly responsive to treatment, including acute leukaemia and lymphoma. This component also addresses rehabilitation aimed at improving the quality of life of patients with impairments due to cancer (see Diagnosis and Treatment module).

Palliative care meets the needs of all patients requiring relief from symptoms, and the needs of patients and their families for psychosocial and supportive care. This is particularly true when patients are in advanced stages and have a very low chance of being cured, or when they are facing the terminal phase of the disease. Because of the emotional, spiritual, social and economic consequences of cancer and its management, palliative care services addressing the needs of patients and their families, from the time of diagnosis, can improve quality of life and the ability to cope effectively (see Palliative Care module).

Despite cancer being a global public health problem, many governments have not yet included cancer control in their health agendas. There are competing health problems, and interventions may be chosen in response to the demands of interest groups, rather than in response to population needs or on the basis of cost-effectiveness and affordability.

Low-income and disadvantaged groups are generally more exposed to avoidable cancer risk factors, such as environmental carcinogens, tobacco use, alcohol abuse and infectious agents. These groups have less political influence, less access to health services, and lack education that can empower them to make decisions to protect and improve their own health.

BASIC PRINCIPLES OF CANCER CONTROL

- **Leadership** to create clarity and unity of purpose, and to encourage team building, broad participation, ownership of the process, continuous learning and mutual recognition of efforts made

- **Involvement of stakeholders** of all related sectors, and at all levels of the decision-making process, to enable active participation and commitment of key players for the benefit of the programme.

- **Creation of partnerships** to enhance effectiveness through mutually beneficial relationships, and build upon trust and complementary capacities of partners from different disciplines and sectors.

- **Responding to the needs of people** at risk of developing cancer or already presenting with the disease, in order to meet their physical, psychosocial and spiritual needs across the full continuum of care.

- **Decision-making** based on evidence, social values and efficient and cost-effective use of resources that benefit the target population in a sustainable and equitable way.

- **Application of a systemic approach** by implementing a comprehensive programme with interrelated key components sharing the same goals and integrated with other related programmes and to the health system.

- **Seeking continuous improvement**, innovation and creativity to maximize performance and to address social and cultural diversity, as well as the needs and challenges presented by a changing environment.

- **Adoption of a stepwise approach** to planning and implementing interventions, based on local considerations and needs. (see next page for WHO stepwise framework for chronic diseases prevention and control, as applied to cancer control).

Series overview
WHO stepwise framework

1 **PLANNING STEP 1**
Where are we now?

Investigate the present state of the cancer problem, and cancer control services or programmes.

2 **PLANNING STEP 2**
Where do we want to be?

Formulate and adopt policy. This includes defining the target population, setting goals and objectives, and deciding on priority interventions across the cancer continuum.

3 **PLANNING STEP 3**
How do we get there?

Identify the steps needed to implement the policy.

The planning phase is followed by the policy implementation phase.

Implementation step 1
CORE

Implement interventions in the policy that are feasible now, with existing resources.

Implementation step 2
EXPANDED

Implement interventions in the policy that are feasible in the medium term, with a realistically projected increase in, or reallocation of, resources.

Implementation step 3
DESIRABLE

Implement interventions in the policy that are beyond the reach of current resources, if and when such resources become available.

PREVENTION MODULE CONTENTS

KEY MESSAGES	2
TAKING ACTION TO PREVENT CANCER	4
CANCER RISK FACTORS	7
PLANNING STEP 1: WHERE ARE WE NOW?	10
How to assess risk factors	11
Use risk assessment to identify priorities for action to prevent cancer	15
PLANNING STEP 2: WHERE DO WE WANT TO BE?	16
What works in prevention?	17
PLANNING STEP 3: HOW DO WE GET THERE?	26
Appoint a focal point	27
Select core risk factors and core interventions	28
Control tobacco use	30
Promote a healthy diet and physical activity and the reduction of overweight and obesity	34
Reduce harmful alcohol use	36
Immunize against hepatitis B virus	38
Prepare to immunize against human papilloma virus	39
Reduce exposure to environmental carcinogens	39
Reduce exposure to occupational carcinogens	41
Reduce exposure to radiation	43
CONCLUSION	45
REFERENCES	46
ACKNOWLEDGEMENTS	48

PREVENTION

KEY MESSAGES

Cancer prevention is an essential component of all cancer control plans because about 40% of all cancer deaths can be prevented.

- Important cancer risk factors – such as tobacco use – are also risk factors for other chronic diseases, including cardiovascular disease and diabetes. Cancer prevention should, therefore, be planned and implemented in the context of other chronic disease prevention programmes, as well as in the context of overall cancer control planning.

- Gender plays a significant role in exposure to risks.

- Many effective interventions to reduce cancer risk are appropriate for resource-constrained settings.

- Activities that are immediately feasible and likely to have the greatest impact for the investment should be selected for implementation first. This is at the heart of a stepwise approach.

- Monitoring trends in cancer risk factors in the population is important for predicting the future cancer burden and for rational decision-making in terms of prioritizing scarce resources.

- A comprehensive surveillance and evaluation system should be an integral element of prevention policies and programmes.

- Regardless of resource level, every country can take steps to curb the cancer epidemic by undertaking primary prevention actions and thereby avoid unnecessary suffering and premature death.

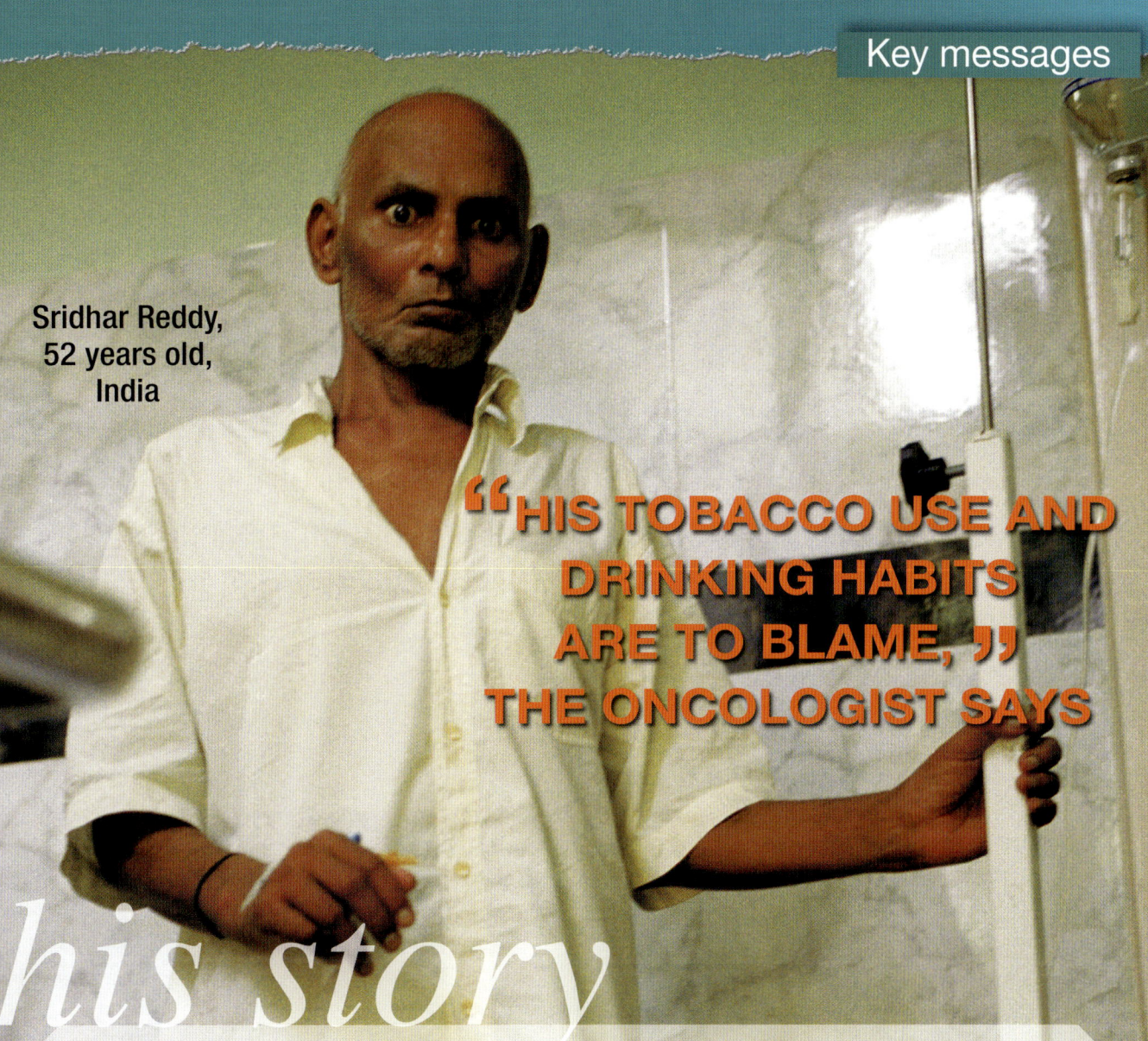

Key messages

Sridhar Reddy,
52 years old,
India

"HIS TOBACCO USE AND DRINKING HABITS ARE TO BLAME," THE ONCOLOGIST SAYS

his story

Like millions of others in 2005, K. Sridhar Reddy died from a cancer that could have been prevented. Still a young man at the age of 52, Sridhar left behind his grieving wife and daughter, and also a substantial debt that was incurred by his treatment costs.

Sridhar chewed tobacco since his teenage years and drank alcohol daily for more than 20 years. "Too much stress," Sridhar explained when the photographer came to visit him in hospital. Sridhar had a first malignant tumour removed from his right check in 2004, and a second one from his throat in 2005. By the time of his interview, his cancer had spread to his lungs and liver.

Despite being cared for at the renowned Chennai Cancer Institute, Sridhar's physicians were powerless to cure him. His cancer was simply too aggressive and sadly, Sridhar died only a short time after he was interviewed.

WHO estimates that 40% of all cancer deaths is preventable. Tobacco use and harmful alcohol use are among the most important risk factors for the disease.

Source: adapted from *Preventing chronic diseases: a vital investment*, World Health Organization, 2005. Photo © WHO/Chris de Bode.

PREVENTION

TAKING ACTION
TO PREVENT CANCER

Cancer prevention is an essential component of the fight against cancer. Unfortunately, many prevention measures that are both cost-effective and inexpensive have yet to be widely implemented in many countries.

Cancer prevention must be considered in the context of activities to prevent other chronic diseases, especially those with which cancer shares common risk factors, such as cardiovascular diseases, diabetes, chronic respiratory diseases and alcohol dependence. Common risk factors underlying all these conditions include:
- tobacco use,
- alcohol use,
- dietary factors including low fruit and vegetable intake,
- physical inactivity,
- overweight and obesity.

Other important cancer risk factors include exposure to:
- physical carcinogens, such as ultraviolet (UV) and ionizing radiation;
- chemical carcinogens, such as benzo(a)pyrene, formaldehyde and aflatoxins (food contaminants), and fibres such as asbestos;
- biological carcinogens, such as infections by viruses, bacteria and parasites.

Interventions aimed at reducing levels of the above risk factors in the population will not only reduce the incidence of cancer but also that of the other conditions that share these risks. Among the most important modifiable risk factors for cancer (Ezzati et al., 2004, Danaei et al., 2005, Driscoll et al., 2005) are:
- tobacco use – responsible for up to 1.5 million cancer deaths per year (60% of these deaths occur in low- and middle-income countries);

- overweight, obesity and physical inactivity – together responsible for 274 000 cancer deaths per year;
- harmful alcohol use – responsible for 351 000 cancer deaths per year;
- sexually transmitted human papilloma virus (HPV) infection – responsible for 235 000 cancer deaths per year;
- air pollution (outdoor and indoor) – responsible for 71 000 cancer deaths per year;
- occupational carcinogens – responsible for at least 152 000 cancer deaths per year.

The prevalence of known cancer risk factors varies in different parts of the world. This is reflected in the proportion of cancer deaths attributable to different risk factors (Figure 1).

Figure 1. Contribution of selected risk factors to all cancer deaths, worldwide, in high-income countries, and in low- and middle-income countries

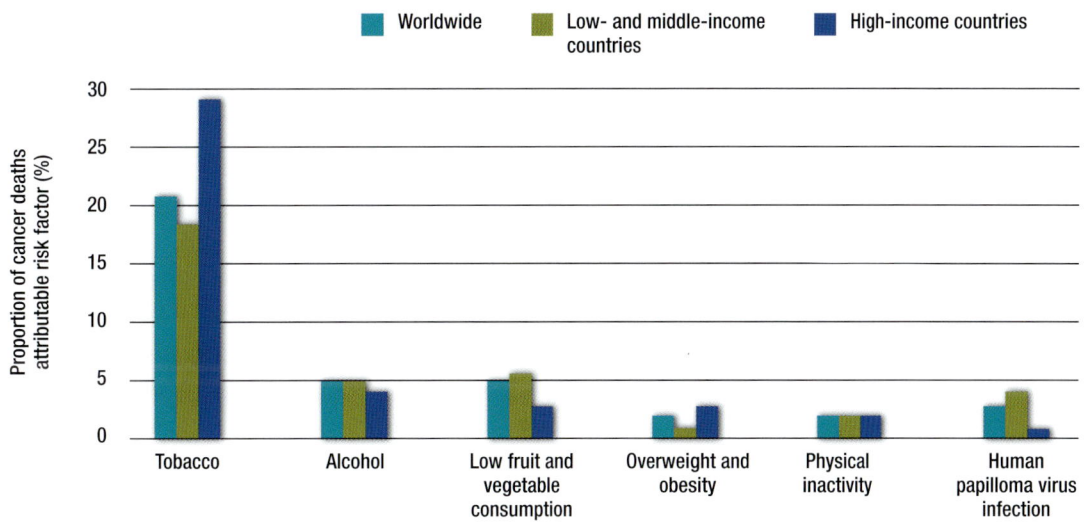

Source: based on data from Danaei et al., 2005.

WHO has proposed a goal of reducing global chronic disease death rates by an additional 2% per annum, over and above projected trends, from 2006 to 2015. Achieving the goal would avoid around 8 million cancer deaths over the next decade. The control of cancer risk factors will have a major role in achieving this goal.

This *Prevention* module first describes the impact of different risk factors on the cancer burden. It then presents the three planning steps of the WHO stepwise framework for preventing chronic diseases (WHO, 2005a) as applied to cancer prevention. These are as follows:

PREVENTION

PLANNING STEP 1:
Where are we now?
Prevention Planning step 1 provides guidance on:
- how to assess the extent of the cancer problem related to single risk factors and to the combined effect of several risk factors (e.g. tobacco and alcohol);
- how to identify the risk factors of major public health relevance in a specific country;
- how to estimate the attributable and avoidable burden related to exposure to the risk factors.

PLANNING STEP 2:
Where do we want to be?
Prevention Planning step 2 gives advice on:
- what can be done – on the basis of currently available knowledge about effective interventions – to achieve a reduction in exposure to cancer risks.

PLANNING STEP 3:
How do we get there?
Prevention Planning step 3 provides:
- advice on how to translate knowledge into practice;
- guidance on how to select interventions in accordance with the resources available;
- examples of best practice in implementing prevention programmes.

Planning needs to be followed by a series of implementation steps. Implementing a chosen set of core interventions will form the basis for further action. Each country should decide on the package of interventions that will constitute the first, core implementation step. This choice should be made according to the country's own priorities and circumstances, including its capacity for implementation, the acceptability of the intervention, and the availability of political and nongovernmental support.

CANCER RISK FACTORS

Major risk factors have a huge impact on the global cancer burden.

TOBACCO, through its various forms of exposure, constitutes the main cause of cancer-related deaths worldwide among men, and increasingly among women. Forms of exposure include active smoking, breathing secondhand tobacco smoke (passive or involuntary smoking) and smokeless tobacco. Tobacco causes a variety of cancer types, such as lung, oesophageal, laryngeal, oral, bladder, kidney, stomach, cervical and colorectal. The total death toll in 2005 from tobacco use was estimated at 5.4 million people (Mathers & Loncar, 2006), including about 1.5 million cancer deaths. If present usage patterns continue, the overall number of tobacco-related deaths is projected to rise to about 6.4 million in 2015, including 2.1 million cancer deaths. In 2030, the projected overall death toll will amount to 8.3 million. In low- and middle-income countries, tobacco attributable deaths have been projected to double between 2002 and 2030.

PHYSICAL INACTIVITY, DIETARY FACTORS, OBESITY AND BEING OVERWEIGHT play an important role as causes of cancer. These factors are affected by gender norms. Because all these factors are intimately interconnected at the individual and contextual levels, estimating the specific contribution of each of these risk factors is difficult and might underestimate the cumulative potential risk.

Overweight and obesity are causally associated with several common cancer types, including cancers of the oesophagus, colorectum, breast in postmenopausal women, endometrium and kidney (WHO, 2003a).

Physical inactivity is a major contributor to the rise in rates of overweight and obesity in many parts of the world, and independently increases the risk of some cancers. Taken together, raised body mass index and physical inactivity account for an attributable fraction of 19% of breast cancer mortality, and 26% of colorectal cancer mortality (Danaei et al., 2005). Overweight and obesity alone account for 40% of endometrial (uterus) cancer. Overweight, obesity and physical inactivity collectively account for an estimated 159 000 colon and rectum cancer deaths per year, and 88 000 breast cancer deaths per year.

PREVENTION

ALCOHOL USE is a risk factor for many cancer types including cancer of the oral cavity, pharynx, larynx, oesophagus, liver, colorectum and breast. Risk of cancer increases with the amount of alcohol consumed. The risk from heavy drinking for several cancer types (e.g. oral cavity, pharynx, larynx and oesophagus) substantially increases if the person is also a heavy smoker. Attributable fractions vary between men and women for certain types of alcohol-related cancer, mainly because of differences in average levels of consumption. For example, 22% of mouth and oropharynx cancers in men are attributable to alcohol whereas in women the attributable burden drops to 9%. A similar sex difference exists for oesophageal and liver cancers (Rehm et al., 2004).

Chronic HEPATITIS B VIRUS (HBV) infection (chronic hepatitis) causes about 52% of the world's hepatocellular carcinomas, resulting in nearly 340 000 deaths per year (Perz et al 2006). Another 20% of hepatocellular cancers (124 000 deaths) are caused by **hepatitis C virus (HCV)** infection. HBV infections interact with exposure to aflatoxin (through consumption of contaminated food) in increasing the risk of liver cancer. Both HBV infections and exposure to aflatoxin are particularly common in sub-Saharan Africa and some parts of south-east Asia, and are believed to be the cause of up to 80% of liver cancer cases that occur in these regions (IARC/WHO, 2003).

HUMAN PAPILLOMA VIRUS (HPV) is the world's most common sexually transmitted viral infection of the reproductive tract, infecting an estimated 660 million people per year. It is also estimated to cause almost all cases of cervical cancer, 90% of anal cancers and 40% of cancers of the external genitalia. HPV also causes cancer of the oral cavity and the oropharynx. Of the many HPV genotypes, types 16, 18 and more than 10 other types are causal for cervical cancer. The most common high-risk genotypes, 16 and 18, account for about 70% of cervical cancer cases worldwide. There is, however, some regional variation, mainly resulting from differences in prevalence of HPV type 18 (WHO, 2006a).

ENVIRONMENTAL POLLUTION of air, water and soil with carcinogenic chemicals accounts for 1–4% of all cancers (IARC/WHO, 2003). Exposure to carcinogenic chemicals in the environment can occur through drinking water or pollution of indoor and ambient air. In Bangladesh, 5–10% of all cancer deaths in an arsenic-contaminated region were attributable to arsenic exposure (Smith, Lingas & Rahman, 2000). Exposure to carcinogens also occurs via the contamination of food by chemicals, such as aflatoxins or dioxins. Indoor air pollution from coal fires doubles the risk of lung cancer, particularly among non-smoking women (Smith, Mehta & Feuz, 2004). Worldwide, indoor air pollution from domestic coal fires is responsible for approximately 1.5% of all lung cancer deaths. Coal use in households is particularly widespread in Asia.

Risk factors

More than 40 agents, mixtures and exposure circumstances in the working environment are carcinogenic to humans and are classified as OCCUPATIONAL CARCINOGENS (Siemiatycki et al., 2004). That occupational carcinogens are causally related to cancer of the lung, bladder, larynx and skin, leukaemia and nasopharyngeal cancer is well documented. Mesothelioma (cancer of the outer lining of the lung or chest cavity) is to a large extent caused by work-related exposure to asbestos.

Occupational cancers are concentrated among specific groups of the working population, for whom the risk of developing a particular form of cancer may be much higher than for the general population. About 20–30% of the male and 5–20% of the female working-age population (people aged 15–64 years) may have been exposed to lung carcinogens during their working lives, accounting for about 10% of lung cancers worldwide. About 2% of leukaemia cases worldwide are attributable to occupational exposures.

RADIATION is energy emitted in the form of waves or rays. Ionizing radiation removes electrons from material (called ionization) when passing through cells and tissue, leading to cell or tissue injury. Medical X-rays and radiation emitted from natural sources, such as radon gas and radioactive materials, are examples of ionizing radiation.

Ionizing radiation can cause almost any type of cancer, but particularly leukaemia, lung, thyroid and breast cancer. Exposure to natural radiation is largely a result of radon gas in homes, which increases the risk of lung cancer (Darby et al., 2005).

Non-ionizing radiation comprises electromagnetic fields like those emitted by mobile phones or power lines and ultraviolet radiation (mainly from the sun), the latter causing chromosomal damages. Ultraviolet radiation is a recognized cause of skin cancer including malignant melanomas.

While REPRODUCTIVE FACTORS, such as mother's age when she first gives birth, and number of births, affect cancer risk, they are not considered in this module. Decisions on childbirth are usually made in a complex context of societal, familial, and individual perspectives and are not primarily driven by the desire to reduce cancer risk.

The longer women breastfeed the more they are protected against breast cancer (Collaborative Group on Hormonal Factors in Breast Cancer, 2002). WHO is promoting breastfeeding by means of the global strategy for infant and young child feeding (http://www.who.int/nutrition/publications/infantfeeding/en/index.html <http://www.who.int/nutrition/publications/infantfeeding/en/index.html>).

Combined hormonal contraception modifies slightly the risk of some cancers. However, recent reviews have shown that for most healthy women the health benefit clearly exceed the health risk. Some combined hormonal menopausal regimens have been shown to increase cancer risk (http://www.who.int/reproductive- health/family_planning/cocs_hrt.html <http://www.who.int/reproductive-health/family_planning/cocs_hrt.html>).

PREVENTION

PLANNING STEP 1
Where are we now?

The first step in cancer prevention planning is to perform a systematic assessment of cancer risk factors at the country level. The objective of the assessment is to obtain good quality and comparable country-level data. These data are needed to set priorities for evidence-based allocation of scarce resources.

The WHO Global InfoBase Online http://infobase.who.int is a data warehouse with a search engine. It provides both country-reported data (where available), and internationally comparable estimates for risk factors (tobacco use, body mass index, overweight, fruit and vegetable consumption, physical activity, alcohol use) for all chronic diseases including cancer.

The WHO STEPwise approach to Surveillance (STEPS) is a simple, standardized method for collecting, analysing and disseminating data on the established risk factors for chronic diseases in WHO Member States
http://www.who.int/chp/steps/riskfactor/en/index.html

Work is ongoing to create country specific risk factor profiles and other information resources regarding cancer prevention and control. This information is available at
http://www.who.int/cancer/en

Planning step 1

HOW TO ASSESS RISK FACTORS

TOBACCO
Surveillance mechanisms are required to:
- understand tobacco use patterns;
- understand the effects of tobacco use in the country;
- monitor the impact of tobacco control policies.

Information is needed about the prevalence of tobacco use, as well as disability and deaths related to tobacco use. This can be compiled from existing national health surveys or by building tobacco surveillance systems, such as the WHO/United States Centers for Disease Control and Prevention (CDC) Global Tobacco Surveillance System (see http://www.cdc.gov/Tobacco/global/index.htm).

DIET
Data about overweight, obesity, and fruit and vegetable consumption are available from the WHO Global InfoBase Online for many countries. If there are no such national data, information on dietary factors can be obtained through surveys that assess the situation. WHO has produced comprehensive guidance on standard assessment methods (WHO, 1995; WHO, 2000).

PHYSICAL INACTIVITY
Physical activity levels can be measured by using standardized tools. WHO has promoted the development of the Global Physical Activity Questionnaire (GPAQ) (Armstrong & Bull, 2006). Although the level of physical inactivity is difficult to assess in populations, the GPAQ enables estimates to be made within countries. It also allows for comparisons between countries.

The Global Physical Activity Questionnaire (GPAQ) is available at
http://www.who.int/chp/steps/en/

PREVENTION

ALCOHOL

Alcohol consumption is usually assessed in terms of volume (per capita consumption) and consumption patterns. In many countries, official alcohol consumption records are not comprehensive, and therefore estimates of per capita consumption need to take account of both recorded and unrecorded consumption (Babor et al., 2003). It is important to take into consideration home brews and other locally-produced beverages.

Drinking patterns are an important way of assessing the extent of alcohol consumed by individuals or a population. They are also useful in projecting the health and social problems associated with alcohol in that population (Rehm et al., 2004).

Global data on levels of alcohol consumption can be found in the WHO Global Alcohol Database (GAD)
http://www.who.int/nmh/databases/en/
The GAD provides a standardized reference source of information for global epidemiological surveillance of alcohol use, alcohol-related problems and alcohol policies. The database brings together information on the alcohol and health situation in individual countries (country profiles) and, wherever possible, includes trends in alcohol use and related mortality since 1961. Country-specific data on alcohol use are also available through the WHO Global InfoBase
http://infobase.who.int
The WHO Regional Office for Europe also maintains an alcohol database
http://data.euro.who.int/alcohol/

HEPATITIS B VIRUS

Information about the prevalence of HBV is usually available from in-country sources.

Links to WHO data sources on the hepatitis B virus include:
- Data about hepatitis
http://www.who.int/csr/disease/hepatitis/HepatitisB_whocdscsrlyo2002_2.pdf
- Immunization coverage globally
http://www.who.int/immunization_monitoring/data/GlobalImmunizationData.pdf
- Immunization coverage by country
http://www.who.int/whr/2005/annex/annexe7_en.pdf

Planning step 1

HUMAN PAPILLOMA VIRUS

Data about the prevalence of genital human papilloma virus (HPV) by HPV type and by age group are available for some countries in Africa, Asia, Europe, Latin America and North America (Franceschi et al., 2006). Web-based country specific information about HPV will soon be available through the WHO/ICO Information Centre on HPV and Cervical Cancer, at the Catalan Institute of Oncology (ICO), Barcelona, Spain, as a result of a collaborative project between WHO and ICO.

ENVIRONMENTAL CARCINOGENS

The assessment of environmental carcinogens in a country should start with identifying potential cancer-inducing agents, by reviewing imported, produced and marketed chemicals. Direct exposure to the identified chemicals can then be estimated by examining patterns of use by the population at the source of exposure (i.e. water, air, food). The exposure of women to indoor air pollution should also be assessed. Indirect exposure assessments can be made through measurements of sources of environmental pollution, including specific industries and waste incineration, which release chemicals that pollute the environment (water, air, food).

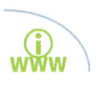

Information about indoor air pollution exposure is available on the WHO web site http://www.who.int/indoorair/en/
The International Agency for Research on Cancer (IARC) maintains a list of carcinogens http://monographs.iarc.fr/
The WHO Global Environment Monitoring System – Food Contamination Monitoring and Assessment Programme (GEMS/Food) provides information on levels of and trends in food contaminants, their contribution to total human exposure and their significance with regard to public health
http://www.who.int/foodsafety/chem/gems/en/

OCCUPATIONAL CARCINOGENS

Assessment of occupational carcinogens includes:

- determining the use of industrial and agricultural carcinogenic substances in the formal and informal workplace;
- estimating the number of workers who come into contact with such substances and are employed in occupations and industries with increased carcinogenic risk.

13

RADIATION

Radiation exposure is of concern:

- in occupational environments (for example, for medical personnel and nuclear industry workers);
- in home environments (for example, radon gas in homes);
- with regard to individual behaviour (for example, UV exposure during extensive outdoor activities or use of sun beds).

Ionizing radiation among occupationally-exposed workers can be assessed through the wearing of individual film badges. National dose registries that collect information on radiation doses among workers monitored for ionizing radiation can supply useful information on occupational radiation exposures, including dose trends over time (UNSCEAR, 2000). Results of surveys of indoor radon levels are available for many countries, including several in Europe (European Commission Joint Research Centre, 2005).

> WHO's UV index indicates the level of solar UV radiation which varies with the geographical location (latitude and elevation) and the time (of the day and year). The UV index is available at
> http://www.who.int/uv/intersunprogramme/activities/uv_index/

JOINT EFFECTS OF RISK FACTORS

Many risk factors act in combination with others. For example, tobacco exacerbates the carcinogenic effects of alcohol use and exposure to asbestos or radiation.

It is important to consider how the cancer burden may change with simultaneous variations of multiple risk factors in a population.

USE RISK ASSESSMENT TO IDENTIFY PRIORITIES FOR ACTION TO PREVENT CANCER

To set evidence-based priorities for cancer prevention, it is critical to know:

- how much of the observed cancer burden is attributable to known, modifiable risk factors;
- how much of the future cancer burden could be avoided through reducing exposure to these risk factors.

The **attributable burden** can be estimated if the past prevalence of population exposure to the risk factor and the relative risk of association with a disease (i.e. a cancer type) are known.

The **avoidable burden** is the burden of disease averted as a result of a reduction in exposure to a risk factor beyond its expected trends. The data inputs required are two exposure scenarios:

- the future burden attributable to risk factor exposure if current trends, health policies, interventions and technological advances remain the same;
- the reduction in burden that could be achieved if risk factor levels were reduced to a lower population distribution.

Decision-making in cancer prevention needs to take into account the fact that risk factors have joint effects in causing cancer and that single risk factors have multiple health consequences beyond cancer, for instance cardiovascular disease and diabetes. The comparative risk assessment project coordinated by WHO in 2000–2001 has produced estimates of the attributable burden of various diseases (including cancer) worldwide and by WHO regions. The estimates give the burden attributable to selected risk factors, taking into account both the joint effects and multiple health outcomes (WHO, 2002; Ezzati et al., 2004).

Guidance on calculating the burden of disease attributable to specific risk factors (for cancer and other diseases) is available for:
- Environmental factors at http://www.who.int/quantifying_ehimpacts/national/en/
- Occupational carcinogens at http://www.who.int/quantifying_ehimpacts/publications/9241591471/en/index.html
- HBV at http://aim.path.org/cocoon/aim/en/vaccines/hepb/assessBurden.pdf

PREVENTION

PLANNING STEP 2
Where do we want to be?

This section gives an overview of what works in cancer prevention. To prioritize actions, knowledge is needed about:

- the extent of the problem (exposure to risk factors and proportion of cancer burden attributable to the risk factors, see pages 11-15);

- the avoidable portion of the future cancer burden (see page 15);

- the effectiveness of interventions (see pages 17-25).

It is also important to consider:

- the social, cultural and political acceptability of interventions;

- the financial resources and political support likely to be available for the planning and implementation of the interventions.

Planning step 2

WHAT WORKS IN PREVENTION?

Broadly speaking, there are two alternative approaches to reducing the risk of cancer:

- to focus interventions on the people most likely to benefit from them because they are at highest risk;
- to try to reduce risks across the entire population, regardless of each individual's risk or potential benefit.

In the overall population, people at high risk for any given condition, including cancer, are in the minority. However, they do not form a distinct group, but are rather part of a continuum across which risk increases. A large number of people exposed to a small risk may generate many more cancer cases than a small number exposed to a high risk. For these reasons, population-wide interventions have the greatest potential for prevention (Rose, 1992). Effective interventions for individuals at high risk exist for certain risk factors (i.e. occupational exposure) and can be combined with population-based interventions to achieve maximal risk reduction.

The following sections outline current knowledge about the effectiveness of interventions in reducing exposure to the various cancer risk factors.

REDUCING TOBACCO USE

A comprehensive mix of interventions is required to efficiently and effectively reduce the risk posed by tobacco products. This mix encompasses interventions aimed at reducing tobacco use, protecting non-smokers from tobacco smoke exposure and regulating tobacco products.

Core provisions of the WHO Framework Convention on Tobacco Control

Demand reduction (Articles 6–14):
- Price and tax measures should be applied to reduce tobacco demand.
- Non-price measures should be implemented to reduce tobacco demand:
  - protection from tobacco smoke exposure,
  - regulation of the contents of tobacco products,
  - regulation of tobacco product disclosures,
  - packaging and labelling of tobacco products,
  - education, communication, training and public awareness,
  - banning tobacco advertising, promotion and sponsorship,
  - demanding reduction measures concerning tobacco dependence and cessation.

Supply reduction (Articles 15–17):
- Illicit trade in tobacco products should be curtailed.
- Sales to and by minors should be prohibited.
- Support for economically viable alternative activities should be provided.

Mechanisms for technical cooperation (Articles 22 and 26):
- Resources available for tobacco control activities should be mobilized, especially for the benefit of low- and middle-income countries, including countries with economies in transition.
- Cooperation should be promoted in the scientific, technical and legal fields in order to strengthen national tobacco control, particularly in low- and middle-income countries, including countries with economies in transition.

Information on the WHO Framework Convention on Tobacco Control is available at http://www.who.int/tobacco/framework.

PREVENTION

There are many cost-effective interventions for tobacco control (World Bank, 1999; WHO, 2004) that can be used in different settings and that will significantly reduce tobacco consumption. The most cost-effective are population-wide policies, including:
- tobacco price increases achieved through raising taxes;
- creating 100% smoke-free environments in all public spaces and workplaces;
- banning direct and indirect tobacco advertising;
- large, clear, explicit health warnings on tobacco packaging.

At the individual level, tobacco cessation is a key element of any tobacco control programme. Working with individual tobacco users to change their behaviour is an important goal, but this will only have a limited impact if environmental factors that promote and support tobacco use are not also addressed.

All these interventions are included in the provisions of the WHO Framework Convention on Tobacco Control, which is an international, legally-binding treaty. As of December 2006, 141 countries and the European Union had ratified the treaty, committing themselves to implementing it nationally. Countries that have not yet ratified the treaty should be encouraged to do so through advocacy aimed at national parliaments and other organizations.

PROMOTING A HEALTHY DIET

A healthy diet is characterized by:
- limiting energy intake from total fat and shifting fat consumption away from saturated fats to unsaturated fats and towards the elimination of *trans*-fatty acids;
- increasing consumption of fruits and vegetables, and legumes, whole grains and nuts;
- limiting intake of free sugars;
- limiting salt (sodium) consumption from all sources and ensuring that salt is iodized.

Specific dietary recommendations for cancer prevention are (WHO, 2003a):
- limiting consumption of Chinese-style fermented salted fish, especially during childhood;
- minimizing exposure to aflatoxins in food;
- avoiding consumption of food and drinks that are very hot in temperature.

Effective ways to promote a healthy diet at population and individual levels include:
- financial incentives to buy fruit and vegetables;
- clear nutritional labels on food products;
- providing healthy meals in schools, workplaces and other institutions;
- access to personalized nutritional advice as part of health-care services.

Activities promoting a healthy diet are most likely to be effective if they use a multi-stakeholder approach, are culturally appropriate and provide information about energy balance and the important role of physical activity.

The WHO Global Strategy on Diet, Physical Activity and Health (WHA57.17) provides a comprehensive set of policy recommendations:
- concerning the environment;
- aimed at individual behavioural changes;
- addressing the food and non-alcoholic beverage industries;
- encouraging environmental planning to promote increased physical activity.

More information on diet and physical activity is available at
http://www.who.int/dietphysicalactivity/en/

INCREASING REGULAR PHYSICAL ACTIVITY

To increase physical activity levels in a population, it is necessary to adopt an integrated approach involving not only the health sector, but also the sport and recreation, education, transport and urban planning sectors.

When planning cities and residential areas, national and provincial governments need to ensure that facilities and services are available for physical activity. Transport policies should encourage walking and cycling, and discourage the use of cars.

Changing the built environment can lead to increased levels of physical activity. Rates of walking and cycling are increased in communities with high population densities, mixed land use and well-constructed interconnected footpaths, relative to those in low density neighbourhoods, typical of urban sprawl. Programmes promoting car-free days and encouraging walking and cycling by closing city streets to traffic have shown good public participation. Transit-type transport systems involving walking and a train or bus ride support increased physical activity levels more so than transport systems that are heavily reliant on motor cars.

PREVENTION

In some cultures, it may be necessary to have gender-sensitive policies and provide places where women can exercise in a "sheltered" environment. In many cities, there may also be a need to improve security (e.g. better lighting, properly maintained footpaths and cycle tracks) so people can walk or cycle to work in safety.

Most interventions targeting individuals are effective in producing short-term changes in physical activity levels and are likely to be effective in producing mid- to long-term changes. Interventions promoting moderate intensity activity, particularly walking, which are not facility dependent, are also associated with longer-term changes in behaviour. Brief advice from a health professional, supported by written materials, is likely to be effective in producing a modest, short-term effect on physical activity but referral to a community-based exercise specialist can lead to longer-term (> 8 months) changes in physical activity.

WHO Member States have agreed to celebrate "Move for Health" Day annually to promote physical activity. This campaign aims to increase regular physical activity among men and women of all ages and conditions, in all domains (leisure, transport, work) and in all settings (school, community, home, workplace).

For more information on Move for Health visit
http://www.who.int/moveforhealth/en/

REDUCING OVERWEIGHT AND OBESITY

WHO recommends that people maintain a healthy weight throughout their lives. The body mass index (BMI) is a simple index of weight-for-height commonly used to define healthy weight ranges in adult populations (for more information see box).

Body mass index

Body mass index (BMI) is defined as weight in kilograms divided by the square of the height in metres (kg/m^2). It provides the most useful population-level measure of overweight and obesity as it is the same for both sexes and for all ages of adults. However, it should be considered as a rough guide because it may not correspond to the same degree of fatness in different individuals.

WHO defines "overweight" as a BMI equal to or more than 25, and "obesity" as a BMI equal to or more than 30. These cut-off points provide a benchmark for individual assessment, but there is evidence that risk of chronic disease in populations increases progressively from a BMI of 21.

Strategies to reduce overweight and obesity must combine interventions aimed at both a healthy diet and physical activity (see above). The causes of overweight and obesity are multifactorial, so the strategies need to be comprehensive and multisectoral in their approach, and to be implemented in a variety of settings (community, workplace, schools, and health-care settings) (WHO, 2005a). In some countries, it may also be necessary to campaign to change cultural perceptions that obesity is a sign of health, affluence and beauty.

No country has yet been able to slow down or stop the epidemic of overweight and obesity. Evidence to date supports preventive interventions encouraging physical activity and a healthy diet while restricting sedentary activities and offering behavioural support. These interventions should involve the whole family, schools and the wider community (Doak, 2002).

Preventing obesity in children and young people is an important priority. Evidence exists that school-based interventions to promote physical activity and improve diet are effective in controlling weight gain among schoolchildren (Doak et al., 2006).

REDUCING ALCOHOL CONSUMPTION

Several effective polices and strategies to reduce alcohol consumption have been identified. Some of the most effective are population-level interventions, including:
- pricing and taxation;
- minimum age for legal purchase of alcohol;
- restrictions on hours or days of sale;
- drink-driving laws.

Effective individual approaches include screening and brief interventions for people using alcohol at hazardous or harmful levels.

The acceptability and effectiveness of these interventions will depend on:
- attitudes of politicians and policy-makers towards alcohol and alcohol-related problems;
- dependence of government on the alcohol trade for tax income;
- prevalence of unrecorded production;
- patterns of alcohol use in different segments of the population;
- perceptions about potential benefits of alcohol in the population.

Based on these considerations, it is recommended that countries use a combination of population-based and individual approaches to reduce the overall volume of alcohol consumption and its negative health and social consequences.

In 2005, the World Health Assembly, in resolution WHA58.26 on "Public-health problems caused by harmful use of alcohol" urged countries to develop, implement and evaluate effective strategies to reduce the health and social problems associated with alcohol.

PREVENTION

REDUCING THE PREVALENCE OF HEPATITIS B VIRUS INFECTION

The most cost-effective strategy for preventing primary liver cancer is universal vaccination with the hepatitis B vaccine. Vaccination strategies are based on the epidemiology of hepatitis B virus (HBV) infections. The development of chronic HBV infection is inversely related to age of infection. Approximately 90% of people infected perinatally develop chronic HBV infection, as compared with 30% infected in early childhood and 6% infected after 5 years of age.

WHO recommends universal infant immunization by incorporating hepatitis B vaccination in national infant immunization programmes, using one of three recommended schedules. So far, more than 150 countries have incorporated the vaccine into their national immunization programmes and several have plans to introduce it in the near future. In countries where a high proportion of chronic HBV infection is acquired perinatally, a schedule providing the first hepatitis B vaccine dose as soon as possible after birth (<24 hours) should be adopted. Consideration should be given to catch-up vaccination of young children and to vaccination of adolescents and high-risk adults.

Important non-vaccination strategies include implementation of safe injection and infection control practices in all health-care services to reduce both HBV and hepatitis C virus transmission. Various behaviour change strategies targeting unsafe injection practices and high-risk sexual practices should also be implemented.

REDUCING THE PREVALENCE OF HUMAN PAPILLOMA VIRUS INFECTION

Condom use offers partial protection against human papilloma virus (HPV) infection. Consistent and correct condom use has been shown to reduce the risk of cervical precancerous lesions and cervical cancer.

Vaccines against HPV infections represent another tool to reduce the incidence of cervical cancer. HPV vaccines have shown excellent protection against new and persistent HPV infections and against moderate and severe precancerous cervical lesions attributable to the HPV genotypes (HPV 16 and 18) that cause about 70% of all cervical cancers.

By early 2007, one HPV vaccine was licensed in more than 70 countries and a second vaccine was submitted for review by vaccine regulatory authorities in the United States and Europe.

Many countries may choose young pre-adolescent girls as the primary target group for vaccination, but decisions of this nature may vary according to local epidemiology and sociocultural settings. The upper age range to include in the programme would depend on the local age-specific infection rates (WHO, 2006; WHO, 2007).

REDUCING EXPOSURE TO ENVIRONMENTAL CARCINOGENS

Cancer caused by chemicals in the environment can be prevented by removing exposure to them. For example, cancer caused by arsenic in drinking water in China (Province of Taiwan) is decreasing after the introduction of measures to reduce arsenic concentrations in water supplies (Yang et al., 2005).

The following strategies for reducing exposure to carcinogens are known to be effective:

- establishing a legislative framework for identifying chemically-induced cancer and eliminating or reducing exposure to carcinogenic chemicals, including the phasing out of replaceable processes or chemicals, decreasing concentration of carcinogenic impurities in products, and regulating drinking water quality;

- disseminating information and raising awareness (by governmental agencies responsible for chemicals and industries, industrial organizations, labour unions and consumer organizations) in forms appropriate for the specific audience;

- increasing access to existing sources of information, such as the International Chemical Safety Card (http://www.who.int/ipcs/en/).

The following international treaties and agreements aim to protect the human and workplace environment from exposure to carcinogens:
- The Basel Convention http://www.basel.int/about.html
- The Rotterdam Convention http://www.pic.int/
- The Strategic Approach to International Chemicals Management http://www.chem.unep.ch/saicm
- ILO Occupational Cancer Convention No 139 http://www.ilo.org/ilolex/english/convdisp2.htm

In countries where aflatoxins contaminate food (mainly via groundnuts and maize), agricultural interventions are required to modify harvesting and storage methods (Turner et al., 2005).

REDUCING EXPOSURE TO OCCUPATIONAL CARCINOGENS

Preventing occupational cancer relies heavily on legislation, regulatory control of the use of known carcinogens in the workplace, systematic assessment of the carcinogenic risk of workplaces and work processes, substitution of carcinogens with less dangerous chemicals, and technical measures to reduce human exposure.

PREVENTION

The effectiveness of preventive measures for occupational cancer follows a well-established hierarchy:

- Reducing use of carcinogenic substances in the workplace by replacing them with less dangerous substances is the most efficient measure. If replacement is not possible, measures to avoid or reduce exposure of workers to carcinogenic hazards can be taken, usually through capsulation and closed processes in which carcinogens are not released into the working environment.

- If exposure to carcinogens cannot be eliminated, it is necessary to control the amount of carcinogens in the working environment, based on threshold limit values established by the competent national authority.

- Finally, when it is not possible to ensure that exposure is within the acceptable limits, workers must be provided with personal protective equipment for carrying out work associated with increased risk.

- In some cases, it is necessary to organize health surveillance of workers aimed at detecting occupationally-induced cancers at an early stage. However, for many occupationally-induced cancers, especially lung cancer, there is no evidence that such interventions are effective.

REDUCING EXPOSURE TO RADIATION

Radiation is an inescapable fact of everyday life and is used for many purposes. Nevertheless, exposure to ionizing and non-ionizing radiation can be reduced by applying appropriate protection measures (ICRP, 1991; Matthes, Bernhardt & McKinlay, 1999).

Ionizing radiation exposures in particular should always be kept as low as reasonably achievable. Dose limits should be respected. These are:
- for the public, 1 mSv/year;
- for occupationally exposed persons, 20 mSv/year.

A large part of the population exposure to ionizing radiation comes from medical radiation. Ensuring the proper justification for all exposures, as well as high technical standards of medical radiation equipment, are important steps in controlling medical radiation.

Various interventions to decrease indoor radon levels are available (Groves-Kirkby et al., 2006). Approaches aimed at lowering exposures to levels as low as reasonably achievable have been successful in reducing individual and average doses in monitored working populations (UNSCEAR, 2000).

The Sievert (Sv) is a unit of radiation dose that includes information on biological damage caused by radiation.

Planning step 2

Cancer prevention is possible immediately after radiation accidents by swift action to limit or prevent radiation exposure. Prophylactic iodine tablets can protect against thyroid cancer induced by radioactive iodine. Other emergency preventive measures may include nutritional restrictions and relocation.

Implementing international guidelines and regulations is best achieved through an independent national regulatory authority working within a legal framework for radiation protection (ICRP, 1991; IAEA, 1996).

Skin cancer risks from UV radiation can be prevented through sunlight protection measures, such as education programmes focused on vulnerable populations (e.g. children, fair-skinned individuals) which aim to raise awareness about unsafe levels of sunlight exposure and encourage changes in behavioural patterns (WHO, 2003b). WHO recommends that UV protection messages for the public include:
- limiting exposure to the midday sun;
- importance of seeking shade;
- using protective clothing and sunscreen;
- using the UV index to estimate UV radiation levels and increase awareness of hazards especially to children, who are more vulnerable than adults to UV radiation.

WHO has established the International EMF project aimed at evaluating the health impact of electromagnetic fields and providing recommendations to Member States on protection from non-ionizing radiation
http://www.who.int/emf/

PREVENTION

PLANNING STEP 3
How do we get there?

This section gives practical advice on implementing strategies in cancer prevention following a stepwise approach. The designation of interventions as "core", "expanded" or "desirable" by risk factor will depend on the feasibility and likely impact of the chosen interventions in local conditions. Decision-making should also take into account potential constraints and barriers.

Key guiding principles for action are as follows:
- National governments should provide the unifying framework so actions at all levels and by all stakeholders are mutually supportive.
- Multisectoral action is necessary at all stages because many cancer risk factors lie outside the health sector's direct influence.
- Interventions should be integrated as far as possible within existing national health policies, health sector strategies and intersectoral programmes. They should be integral components of both the national cancer control programme and the chronic disease control strategy.

Ethics and cancer prevention

In deciding how to develop and implement public health strategies to prevent cancer, four sets of ethical issues deserve particular attention:

- Decisions about which strategies to pursue and the most effective way to pursue them should be evidence-based. Choices that waste resources are ethically unacceptable.
- In making choices among interventions, the aim should be to ensure a fair distribution of benefits in the target population.

Planning step 3

- Governments and nongovernmental organizations, like health professional associations and national cancer societies, should be encouraged to contribute to the implementation process by integrating risk factor control in their health sector strategies.
- Monitoring implementation and outcomes of prevention interventions must be an integral part of the implementation process.

PLANNING REQUIRES:
- appointment of a focal point;
- selection of:
  - core risk factors;
  - core interventions for each risk factor.

APPOINT A FOCAL POINT

A national focal point should be appointed within the ministry of health mainly to coordinate the government's prevention activities. Its tasks may include:
- mobilizing other ministries and agencies whose work touches on cancer prevention (e.g. finance and treasury, customs and excise, trade and commerce, consumer affairs, agriculture, international trade and foreign affairs, law and justice, labour, transport and public services, education, defence, culture and sports, environment, religion);
- building alliances with civil societies;
- enhancing public information and advocacy;
- training a core group of advocates and opinion leaders;
- establishing a mechanism to coordinate the implementation of a national plan.

Initial key steps for the focal point would be:
- to build a national plan of action for prevention based on a situation analysis;
- to establish the infrastructure and capacity to implement the action plan.

- **All relevant stakeholders should be involved in the decision-making process (taking particular care to include women, minorities or other particularly vulnerable groups). The general public should be given access to relevant information about the decision-making process and any conflicts of interest among decision-makers should be clarified.**

- **Some cancer prevention strategies implicitly place collective interests ahead of individual ones. Individual freedom of choice should, however, be protected so it does not compromise public health strategy goals to prevent cancer.**

PREVENTION

SELECT CORE RISK FACTORS AND CORE INTERVENTIONS

Ideally, as many interventions as possible should be implemented to reduce cancer risks in a population. In practice, because of resource constraints, it will be necessary to select the *risk factors* of greatest significance for the country (core risk factors) and *core interventions* to address those risks.

CORE RISK FACTORS

WHO's recommendations include:
- All countries should focus on tobacco control. If they have not already done so, they should ratify the WHO Framework Convention on Tobacco Control and implement the strategies that are part of the Convention.
- All countries should implement the WHO Global Strategy on Diet, Physical Activity and Health.
- All countries should add hepatitis B vaccine to their national immunization programmes.
- All countries should have programmes to control and eliminate the most widespread occupational and environmental carcinogens (e.g. asbestos).

Additional risk factors to be included in the cancer prevention programme will depend on the national burden and priorities.

CORE INTERVENTIONS

A comprehensive approach to cancer prevention requires a range of interventions – from individual to population level – to be implemented in a stepwise manner:
- core,
- expanded,
- desirable.

Activities that are immediately feasible and likely to have the greatest impact for the investment should be selected for implementation first. This is the heart of the stepwise approach. The next step involves expanding the set of interventions. Ultimately, the goal is to add all other desirable interventions.

The recommendations below are not prescriptive because each country must consider a range of factors when deciding on the package of interventions that constitute the first (core) implementation step, including the capacity for implementation, the acceptability of the intervention and the level of political support. Selecting a smaller number of activities and doing them well will likely have more effect than tackling a large number and doing them haphazardly.

Recommended core interventions for each risk factor are summarized in Table 1.

Table 1. Core interventions

Tobacco
○ Raise excise (specific) tobacco taxes to keep up with or outpace inflation and income increases to at least prevent tobacco products from becoming more affordable, and at best make them less affordable.
○ Tax all tobacco products to maintain a comparable price to prevent consumers switching from highly taxed or high priced products to less taxed and lower priced ones.
○ Require by law and enforce 100% smoke-free environments in all indoor workplaces and public places.
○ Ban all advertising, promotion and sponsorship of tobacco products, brands and related trade, including cross-border advertising, promotion and sponsorship.
○ Put health warnings on all tobacco packaging, and ensure that product descriptions, packaging and labelling are in accordance with the provisions of the WHO Framework Convention on Tobacco Control.
○ Establish a national pilot cessation programme in health-care facilities in accordance with available resources.
○ Build media awareness of both the addictive nature of tobacco use and treatment options.
○ Work with appropriate media, in accordance with available resources, to build awareness among key groups, such as health professionals and policy-makers, on the health impact of smoking and exposure to tobacco smoke, and on the relevant tobacco control policies.
Unhealthy diet, physical inactivity, overweight and obesity
○ Develop and implement national dietary guidelines and nutrition policies.
○ Promote educational and information campaigns about reducing salt, sugar and fat consumption and eliminating cooking and preservation methods known to increase cancer risk, for example aflatoxins.
○ Develop and implement national guidelines on physical activity.
○ Implement community-wide campaigns to promote the benefits of physical activity.
○ Promote physical activity in workplaces.
○ Introduce a national chronic disease prevention policy and action plans with specific reference to prevention and control of overweight and obesity.
○ Promote public awareness campaigns about the links between overweight, obesity and cancer, recognizing that an unhealthy diet and physical inactivity are risk factors.
Alcohol
○ Develop and implement an evidence-based national policy aimed at reducing or stabilizing the overall level of alcohol consumption, and link interventions to reduce alcohol problems with activities in other relevant sectors.
○ Raise public awareness, especially among young people, about alcohol-related health risks, including cancer, using gender-specific messages.
○ Promote participation of nongovernmental organizations and relevant stakeholders in reducing alcohol problems.

PREVENTION

Hepatitis B virus (HBV)
○ Implement universal infant immunization using one of the recommended immunization schedules, based on epidemiological needs and programmatic considerations.
Environmental exposure to carcinogens
○ Stop using all forms of asbestos.
○ Provide safe drinking water.
○ Reduce the use of biomass and coal for heating and cooking at home, and promote use of clean burning and efficient stoves.
○ Implement food safety systems (i.e. legislation and monitoring) focusing on key contaminants.
Occupational exposure to carcinogens
○ Develop regulatory standards and enforce control of the use of known carcinogens in the workplace.
○ Avoid introducing known carcinogens into the workplace.
○ Include occupational cancer in the national list of occupational diseases.
○ Identify workers, workplaces and worksites with exposure to carcinogens.
Radiation
○ Provide information about sources and effects of all types of radiation.
○ Establish national radiation protection standards (using internationally available guidelines).
○ Ensure regular safety training of radiation workers.
○ Establish technical guidelines for radiation sources, medical and industrial equipment.
○ Promote UV risk awareness and UV protection actions (including for industrial applications).

CONTROL TOBACCO USE

No tobacco control programme can be effectively implemented without an adequately funded and appropriate infrastructure. Even in small countries at least one full-time employee (more for larger countries) should conduct planning, programming and coordinating activities to design and implement a national action plan. The various elements to be considered for inclusion in the national plan are outlined in the WHO Framework Convention on Tobacco Control. A guide to prioritizing actions and policies is provided in Table 2.

If the country has not ratified the WHO Framework Convention on Tobacco Control, every effort should be made to incorporate strategies for its ratification in the action plan. WHO strongly urges its Member States not to engage with the tobacco industry when designing, implementing and evaluating tobacco control action plans.

Planning step 3

Whatever the situation and characteristics of a country, a basic tobacco control programme should concentrate on implementing at least the core measures set out in Table 2. These include measures related to fiscal policy; smoke-free policies; tobacco advertising, promotion and sponsorship; labelling and packaging of tobacco products; treatment of tobacco dependence; and public education on the addictive nature of tobacco and on treatment options. Treatment of tobacco dependence can encompass a variety of interventions from opportunistic counselling to prescription of anti-smoking medications. Once reasonable success is attained, tobacco control should concentrate on adding other "expanded" and "desirable" measures in these policy areas and on expanding activities to other areas, including regulating contents and sales of tobacco products, liability and litigation (see Box for an example).

A set of interventions to reduce the prevalence of tobacco use is listed in Table 2.

BRAZIL
Prevention in action: comprehensive policies of the national tobacco control programme

- An effective network of national, state and municipal health offices in Brazil has ensured execution of the comprehensive national tobacco control programme. The Ministry of Health shares programme management with all 26 states, the federal district and more than 3 500 municipalities.
- A comprehensive ban on all tobacco advertising and promotion has been implemented, allowing advertising only at points of sale.
- Cigarette packages carry strong visual health warnings and hotline numbers for smokers to seek cessation support.
- Specialized smoking-cessation centres have been established. Training is provided to health-care providers, who deliver brief smoking-cessation interventions in routine work, as well as behavioural aids and pharmacotherapy.
- A specialized agency Agência Nacional de Vigilância Sanitária (ANVISA) has been established to regulate, control and inspect tobacco products.

Source: http://www.anvisa.gov.br/eng/tobacco/imdex.htm, accessed 1 March 2007.

Information on tobacco cessation interventions are available at
http://www.who.int/tobacco/research/cessation/en/index.html
http://www.treatobacco.net/home/home.cfm

To monitor programme implementation, see the following resources:
WHO provides comprehensive tools to monitor tobacco control interventions and policies at
http://www.who.int/tobacco/resources/publications/tobaccocontrol_handbook/en/
WHO annually monitors the implementation of tobacco control policies. The results will be published in the WHO Global Tobacco Control Report at
http://www.who.int/tobacco/en/

PREVENTION

Table 2. Stepwise approach to tobacco control

Policy area	Core	Expanded	Desirable
Fiscal policy (price/taxes)	○ Raise excise (specific) tobacco taxes to keep up with or outpace inflation and income increases to at least prevent tobacco products from becoming more affordable, and at best make them less affordable ○ Tax all tobacco products to maintain a comparable price to prevent consumers switching from highly taxed or high priced products to less taxed and lower priced ones	○ Earmark or designate revenue from tobacco taxes for tobacco control policies and programmes	○ Prohibit or restrict, as appropriate, sales to or import by international travellers of tax-free and duty-free tobacco products
Smoke-free environments	○ Require by law and enforce 100% smoke-free environments in all indoor workplaces and public places	○ Implement educational strategies to reduce second-hand smoke exposure in the home	
Tobacco advertising, promotion and sponsorship	○ Ban all advertising, promotion and sponsorship of tobacco products, brands and related trade, including cross-border advertising, promotion and sponsorship	○ Prohibit display of tobacco products at points of sale	○ Ban youth campaigns to prevent tobacco use if directed, sponsored or encouraged by the tobacco industry
Labelling and packaging of tobacco products	○ Put health warnings on all tobacco packaging, and ensure product descriptions, packaging and labelling are in accordance with the provisions of the WHO Framework Convention on Tobacco Control	○ Prohibit packages carrying information on amount or concentration of constituents and emissions of tobacco products, as measured by the ISO or similar methods ○ Prohibit brand family extensions, for example, through colour schemes, or other identifying names or features, in packages within the same brand ○ Ban any product information provided inside or with the tobacco product package, except government-approved complementary information or warnings relevant for tobacco control	○ Require plain packaging with warnings and toll-free telephone number to help smokers quit

Planning step 3

Policy area	Core	Expanded	Desirable
Treatment of tobacco dependence	o Establish a national pilot cessation programme in health-care facilities in accordance with available resources o Build media awareness both of the addictive nature of tobacco use, and of treatment options	o Integrate tobacco dependence treatment into other disease and health promotion programmes o Train primary health-care providers to deliver effective treatment in various settings o Promote government legislation and incentive programmes for employers to implement workplace cessation programmes o Develop accessible helpline or quit-support services	o Implement community and national cessation programmes o Negotiate low prices for nicotine replacement therapy and other pharmacological aids o Encourage health-care purchasers to contribute to paying for cessation treatment
Public education through media	o Work with appropriate media, in accordance with available resources, to build awareness among key groups, such as health professionals and policy-makers, on the health impact of smoking and exposure to tobacco smoke, and on the relevant tobacco control policies	o Use paid media or media advocacy to build public awareness of the health impact of smoking and exposure to tobacco smoke, and of relevant tobacco control policies	

PREVENTION

PROMOTE A HEALTHY DIET AND PHYSICAL ACTIVITY AND THE REDUCTION OF OVERWEIGHT AND OBESITY

Countries should ensure that they have a national food and nutrition action plan and food-based dietary guidelines.

The FAO/WHO Kobe Framework for Promoting Fruit and Vegetable Consumption should be approved at country level
http://www.who.int/dietphysicalactivity/fruit/en/ ; http://www.who.int/dietphysicalactivity/publications/fruit_vegetables_report.pdf
A WHO report gives guidance on diet, nutrition and the prevention of chronic diseases
http://www.who.int/dietphysicalactivity/publications/trs916/download/en/index.html

HEALTHY DIET

In low- and middle-income countries, the consumption of traditional micronutrient-rich food items and food sources should be encouraged to avoid replacement with salty foods and beverages, or foods rich in sugar and fats.

In implementing dietary interventions, partnerships between the public and private sectors (especially food and non-alcoholic beverage industries) are crucial in ensuring that affordable and healthy food choices are available. Partnerships need to include parents, community groups, nongovernmental organizations, industry and the media.

A set of interventions to promote the consumption of a healthy diet is listed in Table 3.

Prevention in action: partnerships for consumption of five portions of fruit and vegetables a day

Programmes promoting the consumption of five or more portions of fruit and vegetables per day have emerged in many countries with support from ministries of health and ministries of agriculture. Activities include providing information through electronic and other media, point-of-sales promotions, education about fruit and vegetables, providing fruit to schoolchildren, and broad social marketing campaigns.

Source: Pomerleau J et al. (2005). *Effectiveness of interventions and programmes promoting fruit and vegetable intake. Background paper for the WHO/FAO workshop on fruit and vegetable promotion* (http://www.who.int/dietphysicalactivity/publications/f&v_promotion_effectiveness.pdf, accessed 1 March 2007).

Table 3. Stepwise approach to promote a healthy diet, physical activity and the reduction of overweight and obesity

Core	Expanded	Desirable
○ Develop and implement national dietary guidelines and nutrition policies ○ Promote education and information campaigns about reducing salt, sugar and fat consumption and eliminating cooking and preservation methods known to increase cancer risk	○ Ensure that all health claims on food labelling have a sound scientific basis ○ Provide economic incentives to increase the availability and affordability of fruit and vegetables ○ Train health-care professionals to give evidence-based advice on a healthy diet ○ Promote a healthy diet in schools, workplaces and hospitals	○ Introduce regulatory controls on marketing of foods and non-alcoholic beverages to children ○ Support further research on dietary habits and cancers
○ Develop and implement national guidelines on physical activity ○ Implement community-wide campaigns to promote the benefits of physical activity ○ Promote physical activity in workplaces	○ Train health professionals to give evidence-based advice on physical activity ○ Develop sport infrastructures and improve access to existing sports facilities ○ Ensure parks and other places are available for recreational physical activity	○ Create fiscal incentives for sport and recreational centres and equipment ○ Develop national transport policy options that encourage forms of active transport
○ Introduce a national chronic disease prevention policy and action plans with specific reference to prevention and control of overweight and obesity ○ Promote public awareness campaigns about the links between overweight, obesity and cancer, recognizing that an unhealthy diet and physical inactivity are risk factors		○ Design, implement and evaluate community and school-based programmes for overweight and obesity prevention ○ Train all health-care professionals to provide counselling on healthy diet, increasing physical activity and options for overweight and obesity treatment in the health-care system ○ Ensure that marketing of food and non-alcoholic beverages does not exploit the inexperience and credulity of children

PREVENTION

PHYSICAL ACTIVITY

The promotion of physical activity should focus on encouraging appropriate transport options, traditional sports, recreational activities and cultural events, as well as activities at home. There are many opportunities for people to be physically active at work (either at their place of employment or at home), in transit and during leisure time. Policies and initiatives must create environments that help people be more physically active. At least 30 minutes of moderate intensity activity each day is recommended to reduce the risk of heart disease, stroke, type II diabetes, and colon and breast cancer.

A set of interventions to promote physical activity is listed in Table 3.

The WHO framework to monitor and evaluate implementation of the Global Strategy on Diet, Physical Activity and Health is available at
http://www.who.int/dietphysicalactivity/Indicators%20paper-%20English%20Version%20-May%202006%20%20.pdf

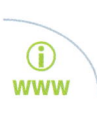

REDUCE HARMFUL ALCOHOL USE

There are several well-tested strategies to reduce harmful alcohol use. These strategies can be applied to a wide variety of settings. A set of interventions to reduce alcohol use is listed in Table 4.

Useful platforms for developing alcohol control measures include:
- WHO guidelines for monitoring alcohol-related harm and an overview of policy options
  http://www.who.int/substance_abuse/en/
- The Framework for Alcohol Policy in the WHO European Region
  http://www.euro.who.int/document/e883.pdf
- The Australian national alcohol strategy
  http://www.alcohol.gov.au/new_strategy.htm

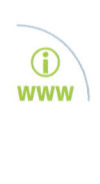

Monitoring the implementation of alcohol policy recommendations is difficult because many different government entities must introduce or enforce these measures. Existing monitoring systems need to be strengthened (or new systems created where they are lacking) so that the effectiveness of policy recommendations at national, regional and global levels can be properly measured and assessed.

Various efforts have been made to monitor the implementation of alcohol policy recommendations, for instance:

- WHO Global Status Report on Alcohol Policy
  http://www.who.int/substance_abuse/publications/alcohol/en/
- WHO European Alcohol Information System
  http://data.euro.who.int/alcohol/
- Alcohol Policy Information System in the United States
  http://www.alcoholpolicy.niaaa.nih.gov/

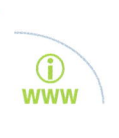

Table 4. Stepwise approach to reduce alcohol consumption

Core	Expanded	Desirable
o Develop and implement an evidence-based national policy aimed at reducing or stabilizing the overall level of alcohol consumption, and link interventions to reduce alcohol problems with activities in other relevant sectors o Raise public awareness, especially among young people, about alcohol-related health risks, including cancer, using gender-specific messages o Promote participation of nongovernmental organizations and relevant stakeholders in reducing alcohol problems	o Revise existing legislation in other sectors to address the need for control of alcohol-related problems o Promote screening for people using alcohol at hazardous or harmful levels and brief interventions in primary care settings o Ensure that people with alcohol use disorders have access to treatment and rehabilitation services o Target high-risk groups and behaviours that are likely to lead to increased harm when combined with alcohol o Encourage formation and maintenance of groups of recovering individuals with alcohol use disorders o Promote training for health-care providers and encourage their active participation in identifying and treating people with alcohol use disorders	o Provide screening for people using alcohol at hazardous or harmful levels and intervention services in health and other sectors (e.g. the workplace, schools) o Make treatment and rehabilitation services affordable o Make young people aware of the risks associated with alcohol by ensuring that education on alcohol use is part of broad health education in schools o Provide a framework for research and information gathering o Develop and maintain a national information system to provide regular data on alcohol consumption and related problems

PREVENTION

IMMUNIZE AGAINST HEPATITIS B VIRUS

Immunization activities against the hepatitis B virus (HBV) can easily be integrated into existing health services. Safe injection and infection control practices should be part of all clinical service delivery.

> The use of hepatitis B vaccines is described in the WHO position statement which can be found at http://www.who.int/immunization/wer7928HepB_July04_position_paper.pdf
> Further references are available at
> http://www.who.int/immunization/HepB_refs_2_Feb_06.pdf

A set of interventions to reduce HBV infection through vaccination is listed in Table 5.

Table 5. Stepwise approach to implement hepatitis B vaccination strategies

Core	Expanded	Desirable

○ Implement universal infant immunization using one of the recommended immunization schedules, based on epidemiological needs and programmatic considerations	○ Provide dose within 24 hours of birth as part of routine immunization (in countries where programmatic considerations have led to adoption of schedules without the birth dose)
	
	○ In countries with low or medium endemicity, provide catch-up vaccinations for older age groups, including adolescents and young adults
		○ Provide additional testing of all pregnant mothers for hepatitis B surface antigen (HBsAg) and offer hepatitis B immune globulin (HBIG) and hepatitis B vaccination at birth for infants of all mothers who are positive for HBsAg
		
		○ Implement routine adult vaccination in high-risk settings such as prisons, sexually transmitted disease clinics, drug treatment centres and as part of needle exchange programmes
		
		○ Provide post-vaccination testing of the following high-risk groups to confirm immune status:
		  - people at risk of occupational exposure
		  - infants born to HBsAg positive mothers
		  - immunocompromised people
		  - sexual partners of HBsAg positive persons
		○ Refer for appropriate follow-up people found not to have protective levels of anti-HBsAg ($\geq$ 10 mIU/ml)

Planning step 3

PREPARE TO IMMUNIZE AGAINST HUMAN PAPILLOMA VIRUS

WHO with partner agencies has developed guidance on preparing to introduce the HPV vaccine and assist countries to decide whether to add the vaccine to the national immunization programme (WHO, 2006). The HPV vaccination will not replace screening and early treatment of cervical cancer.

New delivery strategies must be developed because current WHO routine vaccine programmes mainly target infants aged less than one year (WHO, 2006). Planning and sustainable financing of HPV vaccine programmes need to be considered within the context of comprehensive cervical cancer prevention and control, including screening.

The HPV vaccines are not yet widely available. Where they have been licensed, their current private sector cost is more than US$ 100 per dose (three doses are required to achieve full protection). Manufacturers have declared their willingness to tier prices for countries of different economic settings. Negotiations for tiered pricing and funding sources are needed to make the vaccine affordable in countries of greatest need.

REDUCE EXPOSURE TO ENVIRONMENTAL CARCINOGENS

Preventing chemically-induced cancer at country level requires the following:

- The infrastructure to assess environmental contamination with carcinogens needs to be provided.

- Priorities need to be set so that measures are taken in a systematic fashion and the greatest risks are dealt with first. This requires assessment and monitoring of the levels of exposure to carcinogenic chemicals from the environment (i.e. from ambient and indoor air, drinking water, food).

- Exposure to carcinogenic chemicals needs to be prevented or reduced, for example by:

Prevention in action: reducing indoor air pollution

Several interventions are available to curb indoor air pollution and reduce the associated health burden. The largest reductions in indoor air pollution are achieved by switching from solid fuels to cleaner and more efficient fuels and energy technologies, such as liquefied petroleum gas (LPG), biogas and ethanol or other modern biofuels. In poor rural communities, where access to alternative fuels is limited and solid fuels remains the most practical combustibles, pollution levels can be lowered significantly by using improved stoves with a chimney. These stoves, provided they are adequately designed, installed and maintained, are effective in reducing smoke because of better combustion, lower emission levels, venting smoke through a flue and potentially also shorter cooking times. Evidence shows that women using this kind of stove are at lower risk for lung cancer than women using traditional stoves. The past few decades have witnessed diverse programmes to promote cleaner household energy, ranging from small-scale community-led initiatives to ambitious national programmes, the largest of which has been the installation of some 200 million improved stoves in rural China (see Box on page 40).

Source: WHO (2006). *Fuel for life: household energy and health*. Geneva, World Health Organization.

PREVENTION

- phasing out replaceable processes or chemicals, including removing all forms of asbestos and replacing chlorine-bleaching technology in paper and pulp-production (to avoid dioxin formation and water contamination);
- decreasing the concentration of carcinogenic impurities in products such as benzene in petrol and formaldehyde in particle-board;
- changing processes, for example the destruction of wastes, in such a way so as to prevent the generation of dioxins and furans.

> WHO's Food Safety Department provides scientific advice to Member States, other organizations and the public on all matters related to the safety of food
> http://www.who.int/foodsafety/about/en/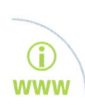

Programme monitoring requires assessment of exposure levels and number of people exposed. Therefore, it will be necessary to use exposure levels to carcinogens and the number of people exposed as indicators of the programme's impact, at least in the short or medium term.

A set of interventions to reduce exposure to environmental carcinogens is listed in Table 6.

CHINA
Prevention in action:
The Chinese Improved Stoves Programme

The Chinese National Improved Stoves Programme is one of the big household energy success stories. In the 1980s and 1990s, the Chinese government implemented the programme in a decentralized fashion, reducing bureaucratic hurdles and speeding up financial payments. A commercialization strategy helped to set up rural energy enterprises; national-level stove challenges generated healthy competition. On the one hand, the central production of critical stove components, such as parts of the combustion chamber, enforced quality control. On the other hand, the modification of general designs ensured that the stove would meet the needs of local users. The programme thus managed to shift societal norms: most biomass stoves now for sale in China are improved stoves. Better stove designs or a switch to liquid fuels could even further reduce indoor air pollution levels and associated cancer risks.

Source: Sinton JE et al. (2004). An assessment of programs to promote improved household stoves in China. *Energy for Sustainable Development*, 8:33–52.

Planning step 3

Table 6. Stepwise approach to reduce exposure to environmental carcinogens

Core	Expanded	Desirable
○ Stop using all forms of asbestos ○ Provide safe drinking water ○ Reduce use of biomass and coal for heating and cooking at home, and promote use of clean burning and efficient stoves ○ Implement food safety systems (i.e. legislation and monitoring) focusing on key contaminants	○ Assess the cancer burden attributable to environmental carcinogens ○ Introduce regulations to restrict trade and use of known human carcinogens ○ Develop and enforce requirements to prevent release into the environment of carcinogens from industrial, transport and agricultural sources ○ Investigate which techniques of preparing traditional, home-cooked foods increase risk of contamination with carcinogens	○ Strengthen national capacities to establish links between cancer morbidity and environmental pollution ○ Develop national environmental health action plans ○ Organize monitoring of persistent organic pollutants and other environmental pollutants with carcinogenic effects ○ Implement efficient food safety systems to control all possible cancer hazards in food and provide concise consumer education material

REDUCE EXPOSURE TO OCCUPATIONAL CARCINOGENS

All working premises and processes with carcinogenic risk should be marked accordingly and the access of non-essential workers to such areas restricted. Those employed at workplaces and in processes with carcinogenic risk should be:

- informed about existing risks;
- trained in the correct use of health and safety protective measures for working with carcinogens.

Legal measures should be introduced to control the importation and domestic use of carcinogenic industrial and agricultural substances, preparations, technologies and industrial processes (Table 7). Use of carcinogenic substances and technologies is gradually becoming restricted in high-income countries. Such substances and technologies are tending to be transferred to low- and middle-income countries where national legislation and its enforcement are weak or non-existent. Therefore, national efforts to prevent occupational cancer in low- or middle-income countries should aim to avoid importing carcinogenic substances and technologies by introducing legal measures to reduce carcinogenic risks in domestic workplaces. Such regulations should stimulate identification of carcinogenic

PREVENTION

ARGENTINA
Prevention in action: Ban on asbestos

Every year doctors in Argentina discover between 50 and 100 new cases of asbestos-related mesothelioma (cancer of the outer lining of the lung or chest cavity). In 1997, the government gave priority to the elimination of asbestos in its national plan for the sound management of chemicals, and established a technical task force on occupational cancer. After five years of public hearings, with the participation of government, workers, industry advocates, environmentalists, clinicians, scientists and consumers, a consensus was reached that asbestos exposure represents an unacceptable risk for both workers and the general population. Asbestos industry groups tried to delay the inclusion of chrysotile (white) asbestos in the proposed list of banned chemicals. However, proponents of an asbestos ban argued that Argentina should provide its people with a level of health protection comparable to that in high-income countries. On 1 January 2003, the mining and import of all forms of asbestos were banned in Argentina.

Source: Rodriguez EJ (2004). Asbestos banned in Argentina. *International Journal of Occupational and Environmental Health*, 10:202–208.

exposures at work and the population at risk, and also promote the development of preventive measures (see example of Argentina).

Health surveillance of workers is not a particularly effective strategy, at least in terms of prevention of new cases of cancer, because of the lack of proven efficacy of screening for many cancers, especially lung cancer.

To monitor programme implementation, the programme levels of exposure and the number of people exposed need to be assessed.

A set of interventions to reduce occupational exposure to carcinogens is listed in Table 7.

Table 7. Stepwise approach to reduce occupational exposure to carcinogens

Core	Expanded	Desirable
○ Develop regulatory standards and enforce control of the use of known carcinogens in the workplace	○ Assess occupational cancer risks	○ Develop programmes for cancer prevention and control in the workplace
○ Avoid introducing known carcinogens into the workplace	○ Introduce integrated management of carcinogenic chemicals	○ Organize registries of occupational exposures to carcinogens and exposed workers
○ Include occupational cancer in the national list of occupational diseases	○ Train workers and managers in controlling occupational carcinogens	○ Conduct assessments for carcinogenic risk of industrial and agricultural chemicals
○ Identify workers, workplaces and worksites with exposure to carcinogens	○ Substitute carcinogens with less hazardous substances	○ Estimate the national occupational burden of disease from carcinogens

Planning step 3

REDUCE EXPOSURE TO RADIATION

Key tasks and interventions for addressing the cancer risk associated with both ionizing and non-ionizing radiation are:

- stringent safety regulations and training for workers in relevant industries and the health sector, including if possible:
  - personal dose monitoring of workers for ionizing radiation;
  - national dose registries (likely to be feasible in high-income countries only);
  - regular technical control of radiation technology used for medical diagnosis or therapy;
  - avoiding inappropriate medical diagnostic X-ray imaging (collaboration with professional associations of radiologists and other physicians is essential for this);

- programmes to reduce residential radon through building modifications in countries where this is a problem;

- in countries with elevated sunlight intensity and with populations of predominantly fair skin type, educational and information campaigns focusing on UV exposure prevention (targeting either the general population or specific subgroups, such as young children and adolescents, outdoor workers or other susceptible populations);

- precautionary measures to limit electromagnetic field exposure of the public, particularly children, mainly deriving from electricity and wireless telecommunications.

A set of interventions to reduce exposure to radiation is listed in Table 8.

Monitoring should include assessing the extent to which interventions were implemented, and to what extent exposure reductions were achieved.

- *Ionizing radiation (medical and occupational).* The existence and application of safety regulations for ionizing radiation, both in the occupational and medical field, should be assessed and updated, if necessary. Dose registries provide the necessary information on numbers of monitored personnel and trends in annual doses.

- *Radon gas.* Various aspects of radon programmes can be monitored, such as the number of houses mitigated. Regular surveys are needed to monitor trends in indoor radon levels.

- *UV exposure.* Regular investigation of the number of people using UV protection would be one option for evaluating the impact of measures to prevent excessive exposure.

Table 8. Stepwise approach to reduce exposure to radiation

Core	Expanded	Desirable
○ Provide information about sources and effects of all types of radiation	○ Implement personal dose monitoring of radiation workers.	○ Organize a national dose registry of radiation workers (ionizing radiation).
○ Establish national radiation protection standards (using internationally available guidelines)	○ Promote radon measurement and mitigation programmes in conjunction with the construction industry in countries where radon is problematic	○ Develop and promote guidelines to ensure appropriate application of medical radiation
○ Ensure regular safety training of radiation workers		
○ Establish technical guidelines for radiation sources, and medical and industrial equipment	○ Introduce regular technical quality control of radiation sources in medicine, research and industry	
○ Promote UV risk awareness and UV protection actions (including for industrial applications)	○ Implement international guidance for sun bed use in countries where they are used	○ Develop and implement school-based programmes on UV protection
		○ Establish, implement and monitor UV protection guidelines for workers

CONCLUSION

About 40% of all cancers are preventable, which means that cancer prevention should be an essential component of all comprehensive cancer control plans. Cancer prevention should also be considered in the context of other prevention programmes because important cancer risk factors – such as tobacco use, unhealthy diet, physical inactivity and obesity – are risks for other chronic diseases.

Finally, cancer prevention efforts should be preceded by a systematic planning process, such as that outlined in the planning module of this series on cancer control.

Many cancer prevention measures are cost-effective and inexpensive to implement. As a starting point, all countries should ratify the WHO Framework Convention on Tobacco Control and implement the strategies that are part of the convention. They should also implement the WHO Global Strategy on Diet, Physical Activity and Health, add the hepatitis B vaccine to their national immunization programmes, and implement programmes to control and eliminate the most widespread occupational and environmental carcinogens.

The stepwise approach recognizes that countries have limited resources and that public health should be chosen on the basis of maximizing the health benefits for the population as a whole. To make sure that resources are used in the most effective way, monitoring is essential both to evaluate the impact of current interventions, and to plan for further expansion.

Every country, regardless of resource level, can take steps to curb the cancer epidemic, save lives and prevent unnecessary suffering.

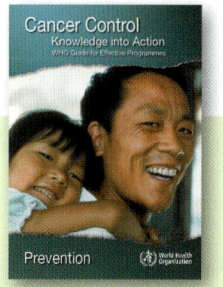

This module on cancer prevention is intended to evolve in response to national needs and experience. WHO welcomes input from countries wishing to share their successes in cancer prevention. WHO also welcomes requests from countries for information relevant to their specific needs. Evidence on the barriers to cancer prevention in country contexts – and the lessons learned in overcoming them – would be especially welcome (contact at http://www.who.int/cancer).

REFERENCES

- Armstrong TP, Bull FB (2006). Development of the World Health Organization Global Physical Activity Questionnaire (GPAQ). *Journal of Public Health*, 14:66–70.

- Babor TF et al. (2003). *Alcohol: no ordinary commodity*. Oxford, Oxford University Press.

- Collaborative Group on Hormonal Factors in Breast Cancer (2002). Breast cancer and breastfeeding: collaborative reanalysis of individual data from 47 epidemiological studies in 30 countries, including 50 302 women with breast cancer and 96 973 women without the disease. *Lancet*, 360: 187–195.

- Danaei G et al. (2005). Causes of cancer in the world: comparative risk assessment of nine behavioural and environmental risk factors. *Lancet*, 366:1784–1793.

- Darby S et al. (2005). Radon in homes and risk of lung cancer: collaborative analysis of individual data from 13 European case-control studies. *British Medical Journal*, 330:223.

- Driscoll T et al. (2005). The global burden of diseases due to occupational carcinogens. *American Journal of Industrial Medicine*, 48:419–431.

- Doak CM (2002). Large-scale interventions and programmes addressing nutrition-related chronic diseases and obesity: examples from 14 countries. *Public Health Nutrition*, 5:275–277.

- Doak CM et al. (2006). The prevention of overweight and obesity in children and adolescents: a review of interventions and programmes. *Obesity Reviews*, 7:111–136.

- Ezzati M et al., eds (2004). *Comparative quantification of health risks: global and regional burden of disease attributable to selected major risk factors*. Geneva, World Health Organization.

- The European Commission Joint Research Centre (2005) (http://radonmapping.jrc.it/index.php?id=37&no_cache=1&dlpath=EU_Reports, accessed 15 January 2007).

- Franceschi S et al. (2006). Variations in the age-specific curves of human papilloma virus prevalence in women worldwide. *International Journal of Cancer*, 119:2677–2684.

- Groves-Kirkby CJ et al. (2006). Radon mitigation in domestic properties and its health implications: a comparison between during-construction and post-construction radon reduction. *Environment International*, 32:435–443.

- IAEA (1996). *International basic safety standards for protection against ionizing radiation and for the safety of radiation sources*. Vienna, International Atomic Energy Agency (Safety Standard Series, No. 115/CD; http://www-ns.iaea.org/standards/documents/default.asp?sub=160, accessed 15 January 2007).

- IARC/WHO (2003). *World cancer report*. Lyon, IARC Press.

- ICRP (1991). *Recommendations of the International Commission on Radiological Protection*. Oxford, Pergamon Press (ICRP Publication, No. 60).

- Mathers CD, Loncar D (2006). Projections of global mortality and burden of disease from 2002 to 2030. *PLoS Medicine*, 3:2011–2030. (http://medicine.plosjournals.org/archive/1549-1676/3/11/pdf/10.1371_journal.pmed.0030442-L.pdf, accessed 15 January 2007).

- Matthes R, Bernhardt JH, McKinlay AF, eds. (1999). *Guidelines on limiting exposure to non-ionizing radiation*. Munich, International Commission on Non-Ionizing Radiation Protection.

- Perz JF et al. (2006) The contribution of hepatitis B virus and hepatitis C virus infections to cirrhosis and primary liver cancer worldwide. *Journal of Hepatology, 45: 529–538.*

- Rehm J et al. (2004). Alcohol use. In: Ezzati M et al., eds. *Comparative quantification of health risks: global and regional burden of disease attributable to selected major risk factors*. Geneva, World Health Organization: 959–1108.

- Rose G (1992). *The strategy of preventive medicine*. Oxford, Oxford University Press.

- Siemiatycki J et al. (2004). Listing occupational carcinogens. *Environmental Health Perspectives*, 112:1447–1459.

- Smith AH, Lingas EO, Rahman M (2000). Contamination of drinking water by arsenic in Bangladesh: a public health emergency. *Bulletin of the World Health Organization*, 78:1093–1103.

- Smith KR, Mehta S, Feuz M (2004). Indoor air pollution from household use of solid fuels. In: Ezzati M et al., eds. *Comparative quantification of health risks: global and regional burden of disease attributable to selected major risk factors*. Geneva, World Health Organization: 1435–1493.

- Turner PC et al. (2005). Reduction in exposure to carcinogenic aflatoxins by postharvest intervention measures in west Africa: a community-based intervention study. *Lancet*, 10:1950–1956.

- UNSCEAR (2000). *Sources and effects of ionizing radiation. Report to the General Assembly, with scientific annexes*. New York, NY, United Nations (http://www.unscear.org/unscear/en/publications/2000_1.html, accessed 15 January 2007).

- WHO (1995). *Physical status: the use and interpretation of anthropometry. Report of a WHO Expert Committee*. Geneva, World Health Organization (WHO Technical Report Series, No. 854).

References

- WHO (2000). *Obesity: preventing and managing the global epidemic. Report of a WHO Consultation.* Geneva, World Health Organization (WHO Technical Report Series, No. 894).

- WHO (2002). *The world health report 2002: reducing risks, promoting healthy life.* Geneva, World Health Organization.

- WHO (2003a). *Diet, nutrition and the prevention of chronic diseases. Report of the Joint WHO/FAO Expert Consultation.* Geneva, World Health Organization (WHO Technical Report Series, No. 916).

- WHO (2003b). *INTERSUN: the Global UV-Project: a guide and compendium.* Geneva, World Health Organization.

- WHO (2004). *Building blocks for tobacco control: a handbook.* Geneva, World Health Organization.

- WHO (2005a). *Preventing chronic diseases: a vital investment.* Geneva, World Health Organization.

- WHO (2006). *Preparing for the introduction of HPV vaccines: policy and programme guidance for countries.* Geneva, World Health Organization.

- WHO (2007). Human papilloma virus and HPV vaccines: technical information for policy makers and health professionals. Geneva, World Health Organization.

- World Bank (1999). *Curbing the epidemic: governments and the economics of tobacco control.* Washington, DC, World Bank (http://www1.worldbank.org/tobacco/, accessed 15 January 2007).

- Yang CY et al. (2005). Bladder cancer mortality reduction after installation of a tap-water supply system in an arsenious-endemic area in southwestern Taiwan. *Environmental Research*, 98:127–132.

PREVENTION

ACKNOWLEDGEMENTS

EXTERNAL EXPERT REVIEWERS

WHO thanks the following external experts for reviewing draft versions of the module. Expert reviewers do not necessarily endorse the full contents of the final version.

Andrew Hall, London School of Hygiene and Tropical Medicine, England
Igor Glasunov, State Research Centre for Preventive Medicine, Russian Federation
Charlotte Paul, University of Otago, New Zealand
Rimma Potemkina, State Research Centre for Preventive Medicine, Russian Federation
Inés Salas, University of Santiago, Chile
Dolores Salas Trejo, Department of Health, Regional Government of Valencia, Spain
Mary-Jane Sneyd, University of Otago, New Zealand

THE FOLLOWING WHO STAFF ALSO REVIEWED DRAFT VERSIONS OF THE MODULE

WHO regional and country offices
Roberto Eduardo del Aguila, WHO Costa Rica Country Office
Jon Andrus, WHO Regional Office for the Americas
Francesco Branca, Regional Office for Europe
Merle Lewis, WHO Regional Office for the Americas
Silvana Luciani, WHO Regional Office for the Americas
Maristela Monteiro, WHO Regional Office for the Americas
Heather Selin, WHO Regional Office for the Americas
Cherian Varghese, WHO India Country Office

WHO headquarters
Robert Beaglehole
Nathalie Broutet
Catherine D'Arcangues
Richard Lessard
Adepeju Olukoya
Serge Resnikoff
Cecilia Sepúlveda

WHO CANCER TECHNICAL GROUP

The members of the WHO Cancer Technical Group and participants in the first and second Cancer Technical Group Meetings (Geneva 7–9 June and Vancouver 27–28 October 2005) provided valuable technical guidance on the framework, development, and content of the overall publication *Cancer control: knowledge into action*.

Baffour Awuah, Komfo Anokye Teaching Hospital, Ghana
Volker Beck, Deutsche Krebsgesellschaft e.V, Germany
Yasmin Bhurgri, Karachi Cancer Registry & Aga Khan University Karachi, Pakistan
Vladimir N. Bogatyrev, Russian Oncological Research Centre, Russian Federation
Heather Bryant, Alberta Cancer Board, Division of Population Health and Information, Canada
Robert Burton, WHO China Country Office, China
Eduardo L. Cazap, Latin-American and Caribbean Society of Medical Oncology, Argentina
Mark Clanton, National Cancer Institute, USA
Margaret Fitch, International Society of Nurses in Cancer Care and Canada, Toronto Sunnybrook Regional Cancer Centre, Canada
Kathleen Foley, Memorial Sloan-Kettering Cancer Center, USA
Leslie S. Given, Centers for Disease Control and Prevention, USA
Nabiha Gueddana, Ministry of Public Health, Tunisia
Anton G.J.M. Hanselaar, Dutch Cancer Society, the Netherlands
Christoffer Johansen, Danish Institute of Cancer Epidemiology, Danish Cancer Society, Denmark
Ian Magrath, International Network for Cancer Treatment and Research, Belgium
Anthony Miller, University of Toronto, Canada
M. Krishnan Nair, Regional Cancer Centre, India

Twalib A. Ngoma, Ocean Road Cancer Institute, United Republic of Tanzania
D. M. Parkin, Clinical Trials Service Unit and Epidemiological Studies Unit, England
Julietta Patnick, NHS Cancer Screening Programmes, England
Paola Pisani, International Agency for Research on Cancer, France
You-Lin Qiao, Cancer Institute, Chinese Academy of Medical Sciences and Peking Union Medical College, China
Eduardo Rosenblatt, International Atomic Energy Agency, Austria
Michael Rosenthal, International Atomic Energy Agency, Austria
Anne Lise Ryel, Norwegian Cancer Society, Norway
Inés Salas, University of Santiago, Chile
Hélène Sancho-Garnier, Centre Val d'Aurelle-Paul Lamarque, France
Hai-Rim Shin, National Cancer Center, Republic of Korea
José Gomes Temporão, Ministry of Health, Brazil

Other Participants
Barry D. Bultz, Tom Baker Cancer Centre and University of Calgary, Canada
Jon F. Kerner, National Cancer Institute, USA
Luiz Antônio Santini Rodrigues da Silva, National Cancer Institute, Brazil

Observers
Benjamin Anderson, Breast Health Center, University of Washington School of Medicine, USA
Maria Stella de Sabata, International Union Against Cancer, Switzerland
Joe Harford, National Cancer Institute, USA
Jo Kennelly, National Cancer Institute of Canada, Canada
Luiz Figueiredo Mathias, National Cancer Institute, Brazil
Les Mery, Public Health Agency of Canada, Canada
Kavita Sarwal, Canadian Strategy for Cancer Control, Canada
Nina Solberg, Norwegian Cancer Society, Norway
Cynthia Vinson, National Cancer Institute, USA